This journal belongs to

_____

My diet starts: _____

and ends: _____

Date ....   Day # ....

Breakfast

Lunch

Dinner

Snacks

Notes

How does my body feel?

Date .... Day # ....

Breakfast

Lunch

Dinner

Snacks

Notes

How does my body feel?

Date _____ Day # _____

| Breakfast | Lunch |

| Dinner |

| Snacks |

Notes

_____

How does my body feel?

_____

_____

Date .... Day # ....

Breakfast

Lunch

Dinner

Snacks

Notes

How does my body feel?

Date .... Day # ....

Breakfast

Lunch

Dinner

Snacks

Notes

How does my body feel?

Date .... Day # ....

Breakfast

Lunch

Dinner

Snacks

Notes

How does my body feel?

Date .... Day # ....

Breakfast

Lunch

Dinner

Snacks

Notes

How does my body feel?

Date .... Day # ....

Breakfast

Lunch

Dinner

Snacks

Notes

How does my body feel?

Date .... Day # ....

Breakfast

Lunch

Dinner

Snacks

Notes

How does my body feel?

Date .... Day # ....

Breakfast

Lunch

Dinner

Snacks

Notes

How does my body feel?

Date .... Day # ....

Breakfast

Lunch

Dinner

Snacks

Notes

How does my body feel?

Date .... Day # ....

Breakfast

Lunch

Dinner

Snacks

Notes

How does my body feel?

Date .... Day # ....

Breakfast

Lunch

Dinner

Snacks

Notes

How does my body feel?

Date _____ Day # _____

Breakfast

Lunch

Dinner

Snacks

Notes

_____

How does my body feel?

_____

_____

Date _____ Day # _____

Breakfast

Lunch

Dinner

Snacks

Notes

_____

How does my body feel?

_____

_____

Date .... Day # ....

Breakfast

Lunch

Dinner

Snacks

Notes

How does my body feel?

Date .... Day # ....

Breakfast

Lunch

Dinner

Snacks

Notes

How does my body feel?

Date .... Day # ....

Breakfast

Lunch

Dinner

Snacks

Notes

How does my body feel?

Date .... Day # ....

Breakfast

Lunch

Dinner

Snacks

Notes

How does my body feel?

Date .... Day # ....

Breakfast

Lunch

Dinner

Snacks

Notes

How does my body feel?

Date .... Day # ....

Breakfast

Lunch

Dinner

Snacks

Notes

How does my body feel?

Date .... Day # ....

Breakfast

Lunch

Dinner

Snacks

Notes

How does my body feel?

Date .... Day # ....

| Breakfast | Lunch |

| Dinner |

| Snacks |

Notes

How does my body feel?

Date .... Day # ....

Breakfast

Lunch

Dinner

Snacks

Notes

How does my body feel?

Date _____ Day # _____

Breakfast

Lunch

Dinner

Snacks

Notes

How does my body feel?

Date .... Day # ....

Breakfast

Lunch

Dinner

Snacks

Notes

How does my body feel?

Date .... Day # ....

Breakfast

Lunch

Dinner

Snacks

Notes

How does my body feel?

Date .... Day # ....

Breakfast	Lunch

Dinner	

Snacks

Notes

How does my body feel?

Date .... Day # ....

Breakfast

Lunch

Dinner

Snacks

Notes

How does my body feel?

Date .... Day # ....

Breakfast

Lunch

Dinner

Snacks

Notes

How does my body feel?

Date _____ Day # _____

| Breakfast | Lunch |

| Dinner |

| Snacks |

Notes

_____

How does my body feel?

_____

_____

Date _____ Day # _____

Today I will reintroduce

Breakfast	Lunch

Dinner	

Snacks

How does my body feel?

Date .... Day # ....

Today I will reintroduce

Breakfast

Lunch

Dinner

Snacks

How does my body feel?

Date .... Day # ....

Today I will reintroduce

Breakfast

Lunch

Dinner

Snacks

How does my body feel?

Date .... Day # ....

Today I will reintroduce

Breakfast

Lunch

Dinner

Snacks

How does my body feel?

Date .... Day # ....

Today I will reintroduce

| Breakfast | Lunch |

| Dinner | |

| Snacks |

How does my body feel?

Date .... Day # ....

Today I will reintroduce

Breakfast	Lunch
Dinner	

Snacks

How does my body feel?

Date .... Day # ....

Today I will reintroduce

Breakfast

Lunch

Dinner

Snacks

How does my body feel?

Date .... Day # ....

Today I will reintroduce

| Breakfast | Lunch |

| Dinner |

| Snacks |

How does my body feel?

Date .... Day # ....

Today I will reintroduce

Breakfast

Lunch

Dinner

Snacks

How does my body feel?

Date .... Day # ....

Today I will reintroduce

Breakfast

Lunch

Dinner

Snacks

How does my body feel?

Date _____ Day # _____

Today I will reintroduce

Breakfast	Lunch

Dinner	

Snacks

How does my body feel?

Date _____ Day # _____

Today I will reintroduce

Breakfast

Lunch

Dinner

Snacks

How does my body feel?

Date _____ Day # _____

Today I will reintroduce

Breakfast

Lunch

Dinner

Snacks

How does my body feel?

Date _____ Day # _____

Today I will reintroduce

_____

Breakfast

Lunch

Dinner

Snacks

How does my body feel?

_____

_____

Date .... Day # ....

Today I will reintroduce

Breakfast

Lunch

Dinner

Snacks

How does my body feel?

Date .... Day # ....

Today I will reintroduce

Breakfast	Lunch

Dinner	

Snacks

How does my body feel?

Date .... Day # ....

Today I will reintroduce

| Breakfast | Lunch |

| Dinner |

| Snacks |

How does my body feel?

Date .... Day # ....

Today I will reintroduce

Breakfast

Lunch

Dinner

Snacks

How does my body feel?

Date _____   Day # _____

Today I will reintroduce

_____

Breakfast	Lunch

Dinner	

Snacks

How does my body feel?

_____

_____

Date .... Day # ....

Today I will reintroduce

| Breakfast | Lunch |

| Dinner |

| Snacks |

How does my body feel?

Date .... Day # ....

Today I will reintroduce

| Breakfast | Lunch |

| Dinner | |

| Snacks |

How does my body feel?

Date .... Day # ....

Today I will reintroduce

Breakfast

Lunch

Dinner

Snacks

How does my body feel?

Date _____ Day # _____

Today I will reintroduce

Breakfast	Lunch

Dinner	

Snacks

How does my body feel?

Date .... Day # ....

Today I will reintroduce

| Breakfast | Lunch |

| Dinner | |

| Snacks |

How does my body feel?

Date .... Day # ....

Today I will reintroduce

Breakfast

Lunch

Dinner

Snacks

How does my body feel?

Date .... Day # ....

Today I will reintroduce

| Breakfast | Lunch |

| Dinner | |

| Snacks |

How does my body feel?

Date .... Day # ....

Today I will reintroduce

Breakfast	Lunch
Dinner	

Snacks

How does my body feel?

Date .... Day # ....

Today I will reintroduce

Breakfast

Lunch

Dinner

Snacks

How does my body feel?

Date .... Day # ....

Today I will reintroduce

Breakfast

Lunch

Dinner

Snacks

How does my body feel?

Date _____ Day # _____

Today I will reintroduce

Breakfast	Lunch

Dinner	

Snacks

How does my body feel?

Date _____ Day # _____

Today I will reintroduce

Breakfast	Lunch

Dinner	

Snacks

How does my body feel?

Foods that are bad for me	Effect on my body

Foods that are bad for me	Effect on my body

Foods that are bad for me	Effect on:

Copyright © Facile Web&Graphic

All rights reserved. No part of this publication may be reproduced, stored in a retrieval system or transmitted in any form or by any means - electronic, mechanical, photocopying, and recording or otherwise - without the prior written permission of the author, except for brief passages quoted by a reviewer in a newspaper or magazine. To perform any of the above is an infringement of copyright law.

facileweb & graphic
showing the world your business

www.facilewebgraphic.com
lucilla@facilewebgraphic.com
Facebook: FacileWebGraphic